# Between The Stones

**Special Thanks**

With gratitude to my writerly tribe: Sam Barbee, Michael Gaspeny, Angell Caudill, John Haugh, Jenny Bates and Sandra Dreis — for your enduring support and creative wisdom.

I am indebted to the Blumenthal family for the shelter and nurture of the Wildacres community, where this book was first imagined. Also to Randy and Sherryl Peters, benefactors of my first writing conference, a blessing I have not forgotten.

# Between The Stones

*poems by*

# Donna Love Wallace

ACKNOWLEDGEMENTS

*Flying South 2019:* "Finishing Touch" (Best in Category, Poetry Prize)

*Medical Literary Messenger:* "On a Summer's Day, Oncology Is," "The Lump"

*Months To Years:* "Voicemail"

*Snapdragon:* "Biopsy Table"

*Westward Quarterly:* "Porch Palm"


Publisher and Editor: Angell Caudill

Copy Editor: Rita Bennett

Cover Design: Pam Fish, www.fishoriginals.com


Author Inquiries and mail orders:
Hermit Feathers Press
3520 St. Leonards Court
Clemmons, NC 27012
U.S.A.

# Table of Contents

*This book is lovingly dedicated to my husband:*

*physician, nurse, housekeeper, comforter*

**the history of my breasts**

       briefer
than life      their brevity my grief
I didn't believe      they would go before me
      they were
not dead      but a bloom of tumors
bound for harvest      from my autumn
      fields
          going to seed

**The Lump**


Doctor 1: *Discovery*

The doctor couldn't unsay it
once he said it —

words shivered out loud
on the coldest November day
condense into cloud.


Doctor 2: *Work-up*

His hands
he didn't know what to do with his hands —
like bees hiving in & out of his pockets.
He sat, stood,
   sat again and introduced himself
   according to the red stitching on his stiff white coat.


*How are you?* I asked.

*I am fine. I'm here to perform your biopsy.*
*The nurse will tell you everything*
*you need to know. I will go now,*
*sign some papers and return.*

Doctor 3: *Diagnosis*

Dead weight of medical terms
collapsing into themselves —
like aging stars
densely dark
clutching all the light they can hold.

## Hardscrabble

In autumn, clay can bear
downy grass from bony

patch. Scrape, sow,
scatter straw. Dance

for rain. Spring cannot claim
every spring-green thing.

# Biopsy Table

Suspicion in suspension —
tissue samples cored moments ago.
Motionless minnows in a jar,
held by a gloved hand, eye-level.
Gloved Hand commands, *Verify,*
*please:*

*Your name? Is this*
*date your birthday?  Confirm*
*today's date and time. Sign here,*
*please.*

Yes, these pieces of me
were extracted today. Take them away
to the lab, lay them under the brightest light, the sharpest eye.
They will say what you need to hear:

*I was born to a woman who bore*
*two daughters. Milk flowed, milk*
*money cannot buy, warmed by a fire*
*no flint can ignite, nothing can douse.*

Outside, a spring snow falls, filling
blossoms on parking lot trees, chilling
the white petals, wilting under the melt and weight.

## The Milk

At the age of four I stepped
outside and retrieved
the dawn delivery:

cold milk
in a thick glass bottle
slick with its own dew.

I learned what happens
when the bottle drops
on a cement porch:

milk escapes,
makes its own
shape. Shattered

fragments rock like boats.
I stand
in the new surging sea.

## Ultrasound

### I

sound
mounds as snow,
a billowing landscape
wakening to the throb and
call of all living
inside these
woods.

### II

leaves
sloughed, dry and
brittle—now silent
and still as cut timber.
bitter whispers shed
from a wizened
throat.

### III

silence
spills, rain-salted,
wrung from blackening
skies, filling my Dead Sea.
I lean in. I float. It
cradles me in
salt.

## Surreality in Food Lion

Modern medicine's Paul Revere approaches me by the blueberry bin.
This self-appointed voice of edible superheroes armed
with magic bullets declares,

*Eat blueberries and you won't get cancer!*

With the confidence of Jonas Salk, the jollity of Santa Claus,
he explains the blueberry's counterattack on free radicals, the culprit
and kryptonite of good health. As he hands out candied advice,

I clutch my cell phone, expecting

biopsy results. It is August, the blueberry harvest abounds. I examine
these tiny round soldiers crowded into cartons, ready to be
dispatched to a bowl of oatmeal or Trojan-horsed in a muffin,

ready to fight, to delay my demise.

My phone quivers, blinks its alert.

## University of Carcinoma

A graduate semester's required reading:
anatomy, genetics, radiation, statistics
    (*humanities,* a footnote).
This eve of exams, sleepless—I barter with deities,
hoping for low grade disease,
the fast track to dismissal.
Every night, I recite
my thesis:
*It's nothing. Nothing.*
*Nothing until it's something.*

## On a Summer's Day, Oncology Is

a farmer's retaining pond of data stocked with
    tadpoles slow growing their legs
under the scum-crud surface, and the percentage chance
    one will jump onto our picnic blanket and
splat your potato salad. However large or small
    the aforesaid amphibian, no matter.
*Invasive* is a word you do not want.

# Check Box

*~ a found poem*

Do your gums bleed when you brush / have you ever had a persistent cough / do you take prescriptions for any conditions / what is this physician treating you for / infections / chest pain / do you have a murmur / artificial limb or prosthesis / if yes please explain / do you take over the counter medication / do you drink alcohol take drugs recreationally / how many times each week do you smoke snuff or chew / are you interested in stopping / do you have high blood pressure chest pain / chronic pain take aspirin / have seizures dry mouth / fainting spells / heartburn / gall stones kidney stones / night sweats skin sores / migraines / sexually transmitted diseases / sinus trouble / trouble sleeping / frequent urination constipation / swelling / dizziness / asthma / anemia hemophilia / are you in good health / check a box below:

YES          NO          DON'T KNOW

have you had cancer / a joint replaced / when was your surgery / are you pregnant / are you positive HIV or have AIDS / hearing aids / wear glasses / do you see a dentist regularly / have glaucoma / have an allergy to drugs latex foods metals / please specify / do you have ulcers / ever had a stroke / do you feel depressed suicidal safe at home / do you take birth control herbal diet supplements hormone replacements / do you have any other physical or mental condition or problem not listed that you think we should know / please know staff is not responsible for any action taken or not taken as a result of errors or omissions made in the completion of this form. Date and sign on the line below:

X

_____

*human forms      pencil-poised      wonder which      will manifest next*

## Surgical Options: Hangnails

*~ for Dr. Lori Kellam*

I look at my hands and the surgeon's hands too. She says, *I see*
    *you have chronic hangnails. We can fix that.*
*We can remove your fingers, replace with titanium digits.*
    I hold the cold, shiny model, examine
the joints, how they hinge. I understand this surgery removes
    the problem, yet requires a new way of grasping things.
*We've been treating this problem for decades with great success.*
    *No chance of recurrence, paper cuts or arthritis.*
I look at my hands, channels of veins filling heart's chambers,
    fingers flush and warm, pulsing, pressed
into my love's palm. Can I part with these fingers?
    How will I feel?

## Decisions

Grasp one of many knives.
See the sunset glint rays
off the beveled blade.
Feel the cool bone handle
pressed in your palm.

Break skin below the sternum,
angle toward your heart carefully
guarded by your ribcage.
Breathe deep and hold. Self-
hypnosis really does work.

Spiral toward the apex,
heart's clenched fist.
Your aim is true if chords of
bass and baritone moan across
cold canyons, reverberate.

Leave the blade in place.
Do not remove. Pulling out will
loose a crimson pool. Button
your still-white shirt. Accommodate
the protruding handle.

Put on a jacket if you must.
Act casual.

## Pre-op Composition

*~ for Dr. Hampton Howell*

The plastic surgeon opens a ring binder of photographs—
cropped nudes of female torsos tucked into clear plastic sleeves.
Privacy laws decree they be headless. I cannot see their eyes.

> They have no hands.
> These parts excised.

The photographer would claim: *This is not a clean frame.*
*Keep the flock whole within the image, cut no*
*a wing or any living thing.*

> Yet I see
> that is the business of this thing.

## Diorama

*~ morning of surgery*

Daybreak penetrates the keepsake
stone illuminating
a dense cobalt knot of storm
trapped inside the core
unable to unleash
upon its heaving sapphire sea
all its fury

**Do This**


Because nothing else can be done,
    do this:
bend your body to the wind.

Let the cold seep in
    the thin cotton weave of
this white shirt. Split

wood, cut no more. Finish
    house chores: dust, sweep. See
how snow-white sheets billow

their one given breath because
    nothing more can
be done.

**felt tip pen**


an artist facing my breasted canvas,
      the surgeon sketches
            hieroglyphics. how alien

the purple pen
      its felt tip
            a dull blade. i am awake.

there is no anesthesia for this
      no medication to help me forget
            plotting this mercy killing.

the hardest thing: enduring
      permanent marker
            charting indelible erasures.
  yet

this sculptor sees her
      new figure conceived,
            chiseled from stone.

**When I Die**

Escort relatives to the next room, so they may wash with tears and change into black. While they do, clothe me in feathers, fur and glittering scales for my return to earth. There is quite a Mardi Gras going on down in the dirt, I understand. Scientists and theologians agree every particle is dancing the rumba.

No choirs, please, just a lit stick of ACME dynamite and a laugh track. Wile E. Coyote's day job was torment, but at the end of the battle, we shared a bottle of champagne and feasted on reruns.

When I walk past cliff's edge, before I know my own falling, before I realize the weight of my ponderous chain, I will breathe the air between cause & effect and wonder about gravity. Road Runner, my resilient hero, and Bugs Bunny, my reliant one, wait for me in downward, distant puffs of dust.

## Near Deaths

All the near deaths life
brings, weeping's mute drip
seeps down into ground water.
Unstoppable, non-negotiable—

yet opposable. Dam its progress,
channel floods to nothingness.
All is impossible, we are not possible,
death more than probable. Like snow,
death falls weightless, filling

small blooms. Winter buries
too soon, all born too late. Breathe,
let's breathe. Let go of spent trees and
dry pools of leaves. Another spring,
somewhere, still runs full stream.

**Voicemail**


His mother said her new oncologist contacted her youngest son—
honest, direct and medically trained— so family knows

she will undergo imaging on the fourteenth of April
and learn results the following week.

His mother said she likes her doctor— he is young,
has two children, and is Brazilian.

*They speak Portuguese in Brazil,* she said,
*but you probably knew that.*

*I know these things because I asked.*
*Don't call back.*

*I'm fine.*

## Wintering Cancer

the hands of the clock tick a litany
once held and loved,
now lost

he kneels by the edge of the tub,
bends to bathe
his wife

who raises her arms out of warm water
and summer rains fall
through her fingers

who knew bare limbs could flower in winter?

## Porch Palm

Pruned & abandoned
time-promised fronds

from this blunt,
leafless stump.

Amputated plant
slanting in rain

leaning in snow
lopsided, exposed

for weeks—nothing
from nothing.

A pledge:
a spear, a rising stalk

stirring shoots
from rooted knot,

a greening birth from
potted earth.

## Bathing Suit Drawer

Pick something.
Put it on. Turn,
check the  mirror.

Pick something else.
Put it on, turn,
look again.

All right? No.
Try another. This?
Last year, it fit.

I have nothing
to wear. Last year,
these scars weren't here.

## Breast Obsessed

gilded vanity mirror
*portrait nude*
glass shower door
*Renoir bather*
boutique dressing room
*Warhol vogue*
shop window mannequins
*no nipples*
travel stop mirror
*peek of cleavage*
subway stairwell
*motion detection*
grocery store cold case
*trapped apparition*
*behind glass*
*stares back*

## Glossary of Size

*Stacked* is just too,
too. . . there must be another
word —

something softer,
less architectural
yet

conveys *gravid*
heft — is *gravidity*
a word?

Yes but, oh
baby, NO.
Let's think.

*Chesty*
is gauche,
*Rubenesque*

fleshy.
Maybe
*pendulous?*

PLEASE NO.
Oh look.
Here it is. . . *avoirdupois,*
   as in
    *she put on a certain avoirdupois like nobody's business.*

## Fitting Opinion

*~ for Beth*

*How big do you want*
*to be?* the architect asks,
waits for the tape measure of
my tongue to unroll and plumb
alphabetical language of brassieres:
A   B    C   D . The golden triangle
breastbone notch, ribcage to ribcage my
topographic map; cartographer's drawings
purpled in before strip-mining begins; shirts
and dresses, my witnesses hanging out in the
closet — we try each other on, comparing our
many  selves each week,  my favorite shirt wraps
herself around  me as I reach  through her sleeves
and  ask,  *Is this all right? Enough? I'm not sure,*
*do buttons pull? Shoulders tight?* Shirt after
shirt, dress after dress — all speak opinions
like best friends and bridesmaids:  yes, no,
maybe so. *I'm still not sure. How the hell*
*do you tell?* Husband says, *Your desire*
*is my desire, it's you I love. Yet yours*
*to decide.*  Then somebody else
comes into my closet: the last
child harbored in this
body, to nurse from
it, cling to it. She
watches me dress,
then suddenly says,
*Yes I can tell, you*
*are  full  enough,*
*because now you*
*look like my mom.*

36

## Girlfriend

Your eyes lower and rise,
over and again, sizing up
The Twins.

Sonar pulsing my curious sea,
imagination mapping
silicon deep.

*A peek?* I offer.
 *A picture worth
 a thousand words.*

A touch, ten thousand.

**Between the Stones**


           Facing the stone fireplace close,
I lower my head, focus on my toes.
           Arms bent at the elbow, my forearms crawl
the rough wall, reaching for the highest rock
                        possible.
                     These arms years ago visited
Jerusalem's Western Wall,
joined shrouded, swaying
           women praying, wedging
                 paper scraps between the stones —
           hand-written petitions entrusted to the holy
       crevices. Many cried for mercy, so much
destroyed by war.

Here, I bear cancer's toll, gauge the pain, pause
           when fingers can travel no further.
           Hands rest
on this rock face. Looking up, I tuck
a white scrap into a thin space.

**Finishing Touch**

*~ for Blueberry*

A strip mall reclines
among rural, rolling hills. Little Vinnie's
Tattoo parlor, lacks a clinical
vibe — pool table, cue sticks,
leather chairs, animal skin rugs.
African ritual masks fix their gaze
toward the hallway where muted voices
hover behind black-curtained doorways.

In the tattoo room, I thumb through
back issues of *Rolling Stone,* then
strip to the waist, unfold a paper drape.
A room of mirrors where art and artifacts
replicate — a horde of animal bones,
sculpture and scrimshaw. The Twins
blend in despite their plain faces,
thin-lipped scars of smile & smirk.

A dozen ink pots like small communion
cups hold hues of blue, blush, tawny brown.
As he mixes a tinted elixir, my desires dissolve.
I tire of all decisions but this: to trust the artist.
*Do you feel anything?* Michelangelo inquires.
Nerves severed, I am numb under the tattoo gun —
only tiny bolts of lightning strike
far below the silicone:

                                    the last
        sensation
                    I will feel
                            so near

## To My Tattoo Artist

*~ for Dr. Susan Hines*

I can't imagine what it's like to be you, Mr. Tat-On-Demand.
Has the Big C backed you into this corner gig —
three shows a day of polka-dot skin tones?

If you went AWOL, we would hunt you down, lock
you in the Prison of Nipple-less Women
waiting to re-enter society. Only you know if

you'd like to mix a fresh palette, create designs for wrists or spines.
Do you miss the muscled expanse of a broad-shouldered man?
The gluteal half-moons of a woman?

When your gig is over, you will rest among the saints.
For you painted frescoes on our Sistine domes,
ennobling our new architecture,

honoring each relic of breast.

## Ode To My Mother's Breasts

My mother was diagnosed with cancer just before I left for a five month hike on the Appalachian Trail. Six weeks into my trip, I came home for her surgery.

My mother, father and I sat on the back porch. They on either end of the long wicker couch and I curled up on the love seat. She told me she was relying on the people in her life and didn't need to see a therapist. It was a genuine remark and I could see that she received the space and time to process this decision from my father and from her friends.

I asked her if she'd said goodbye to her breasts — any poem, or ritual. She told me that she'd been talking to them. The night before she had asked my father, her husband, and the only lover to hold her body, she asked him to kiss them goodbye.

While she spoke somewhat tearfully, my father reached across and brought her hand to his lips. It was the only time I've seen him kiss her so tenderly; the only time I've seen him kiss anything besides her readily-puckered lips.

The night before her surgery we compared our breasts. She let me touch. Ours are the same size. *Enough for you to hold completely in your hand.* That's always the response I receive from lovers when I comment on the small-size of my breasts. They like that they can hold them in their hands.

41

The next morning, my parents attended appointments, pre-op procedures and my mother went under anesthesia. I was out running errands.

In between dropping off my camera film at the drugstore and buying a bottle of wine for a dinner date, I shopped for a bra. I wanted to feel beautiful and presentable. I wasn't able to find more attractive bras among my stored belongings, so I thought I'd buy a cheap black one for the evening.

I made my way between rows of hanging bras. I slid aside hangers with a plastic, grinding click and pressed my fingers to the softly molded cups. Foamy circles inserted in every single one. Years ago I had thrown out all my bras and bought simple, cloth pieces — no padding, smoothing, or lifting. Knowing I would be returning to my travels shortly, and that my date did not truly care, I walked out of the store empty-handed. I had to pick up wine and it was close to the end of mom's surgery.

When I walked into the hospital lobby I looked to the walls and saw large framed photographs of places that I had visited during my travels green mountains, fading into wispy blue ridges. They were familiar scenes, but the colors were overly saturated and mocking. I had just been there. Out there, I carried everything on my back I needed to survive, but now I was here. I headed to the slow moving elevators.

Mom was awake, groggy from the pain medication. Dad stood up from the bedside chair and I walked to take his place. I took my mother's hand. She said with relief - *it's over, I did good.* I told her she did very good. She lifted my hand to her mouth and kissed it with her eyes closed.

There was a slight rise to her chest from the expanders. These would be slowly inflated to stretch her healing skin to make room for the final implants. The surgeon came into the room wearing blue scrubs. Her highlighted hair was pulled back in a loose ponytail. She was so freckled-tan that I couldn't tell the difference between freckles and skin. Her complexion made her blue eyes bluer and I wondered if she went to a tanning bed, or maybe had a beach house she visited each weekend. I followed the freckles down her V-neck scrub top and saw the lifted center of her beige bra, held suspended by the weight of her right breast.

I asked what they do with removed breasts. They dig into the tissue and find all the cancer, they biopsy and test. Then most likely, mom said, they incinerate the tissue. That is the most sanitary procedure. Mom asked about the view from the window. I described a few trees, but mostly rooftops and AC units, and a tall pipe that spewed liquid and steam into the air.

*Probably the remains of my burned boobs*, she said, laughing.

\*   \*   \*   \*

Four days later her humor faded from the narcotic painkillers, constipation, fatigue and emotional struggle. Each day was long and the enormity of the process ahead loomed around every small, quiet moment in the house or on the back porch or during one of our very short walks.

43

It helped to distract her with other projects. We sat on her bed and flipped through magazines. I had a suitcase full. I was working on a project that used hundreds of small pieces for a collage. Mom flipped through the bright, glossy pages and asked me about colors and textures. When I nodded she ripped out the page and placed it next to me.

She stopped on one page. *Those are breast implants,* she said. The picture showed two manicured hands with red painted nails and bulky silver bracelets each holding a clear, round pouch. You could see the red nail polish through the implants, watery and out of focus.

I asked if those were filled with silicone and leaned into the page. The caption offered no helpful information. Mom told me that some implants are filled with a saline solution. Salt and water. Most women choose silicone because it feels more realistic. Her expanders will be filled with saline by the plastic surgeon until they are the right size for her implants.

The article discussed the technology, historical issues and current trends with breast implants. These implants, though were for enhancement, aesthetics, ego, not for cancer survivors. We guessed that in the future regenerative medicine would be able to grow real breasts, tissue and cells, and then attach them to cancer patients. Eventually this technology would become so commonplace that luxury will walk in and models will have home-grown breasts too. She ripped out the page and gave it to me.

It was late and the house was quiet. My mother lay on her back, the only way she was allowed to during recovery. She unzipped her sweater. Underneath was the post-op bra cinched tight with hook-eyes, meant to hold everything in place. There were drain bags for recovery fluid and tubes that were choked beneath the elastic and cotton of the bra. She complained about these tubes.

She unhooked each eyelet and sighed with the release. She moved aside the tubes and drain bags. Her body was bare and exposed from the chest up. She moved her fingers lightly over the tight tape and along the bottom of two white gauze squares placed over her chest. She sighed, enjoying her ability to scratch, ever so slightly, skin with nerves still waking up.

She was so comfortable, half-naked on the bed. Unlike exposing two breasts, real breasts with nipples and hair follicles and sagging weight. She closed her eyes and began to drift off.

I took the picture of two silicone breasts held by red-tipped lady hands and cut it up into small pieces.

*   *   *   *

In the months it took me to complete my 2,200 mile hike and reach Kathadin, Maine, my mom would continue her surgical recovery, complete full reconstructive surgery and even make an appointment with the nation's leading nipple tattoo artist. She resumed her exercise with walking and then hiking and grew to love hiking. One year after I began my Appalachian Trail challenge, and one year after her diagnosis, my mom asked me to take her on a backpacking hike in the North Carolina Mountains.  I couldn't wait to share my favorite outdoor activity. We planned a 3-day, 30 mile trip.

I watched my mother sweat and climb hills with a 25 pound pack.

*"I know this is hard, mom.  We're almost to camp."*

*"I've done hard things before."*

**Donna Love Wallace** of Lewisville, North Carolina, has received Wildacres Artist's Residencies in recognition of dedication to her craft. She has also served in leadership positions with Winston Salem Writers and Poetry in Plain Sight. Her poetry appears in *Snapdragon, Hermit Feathers Review, Flying South, Kakalak, The Paddock Review, Poetry In Plain Sight, Wild Goose Poetry Review, Plainsongs and WestWard Quarterly,* among others. Donna is a retired critical care nurse and seminarian, and recently learned how to brew a lovely cup of coffee out in the middle of nowhere.

CPSIA information can be obtained
at www.ICGtesting.com
Printed in the USA
FFHW021800160919
55033454-60721FF

9 780578 572703